The Superman

Years

The Emotional Life of a Parent Caring for a Child
with Type 1 Diabetes

Linda Rupnow Buzogany, MS
Licensed Professional Counselor

For Jalyn

CONTENTS

Foreword

There is nothing that can turn a life upside down so completely and so swiftly as a major illness. Values we have held, ways we have lived, are all thrown into question as our body copes to survive and to recover. There are some illnesses, however, from which there is no recovery. Though not necessarily life threatening, autoimmune diseases often bring with them far-reaching physical changes for which there may be no cure. Having wrestled with two autoimmune diseases in succession, I am well aware of the terrible hardships they bring in their wake, not only for the one stricken but for friends and family as well. As hard as they are to deal with anytime they occur, they take an especially heavy toll when they strike our children.

Like many autoimmune diseases, diabetes is a life

sentence from which there is still no reprieve. For child and parent alike, diabetes demands changes in how one lives and the discovery and implementation of coping devices. In her book, *The Superman Years,* Linda Rupnow Buzogany discloses the shock with which she and her husband learned of the diagnosis of their young son. In a very poignant and honest manner she allows the reader a glimpse into the turmoil the diagnosis generated in her life and the severe emotional strain endured by her family. Her words and honesty offer real solace for those in a similar situation, who know very well there are no easy answers and no facile solutions to the task fate has given them.

In her down-to-earth and personal style, Linda explains what she and her husband went through during the first difficult years and how, exhausted almost past coping, she was able to hang on and not only find the resources required to care for her son but actually come to see the blessings diabetes can bring along with its travails. She speaks not only of the tasks required on the physical level, but the attitudes that can help one get beyond the shock and despair of finding one's child seriously ill, and the ways to tap one's emotional resources for the strength one didn't know one had.

Equally important, she reveals how she was able to turn to physical and spiritual resources, such as Yoga, to fight the anxiety and exhaustion and to search for deeper meanings in the midst of seeming chaos. By showing the reader the comfort she found in her own dreams she offers an invitation to all to turn to the inner world of dreams where unexpected insights and meanings are to be found. I know that in my seven years of struggling with autoimmune diseases, dreams offered me wisdom and faith I don't think I could have found in any other way. In sharing her story, Linda reveals the ways in which dreams helped her find her way on this difficult and often overwhelming journey. She thereby reveals a dimension to the struggle one doesn't often find when dealing with doctors, medications, and treatment plans. She reminds us that we, and our children, are not only physical beings but spiritual ones as well and that learning to tap our spiritual resources can fend off hopelessness and despair.

Thankfully, Linda never sugarcoats the difficulties a diagnosis of childhood diabetes brings, but allows us to glimpse into the depths of her own struggle. But, however terrible these struggles can be, she also reminds us that they are not insurmountable and that, in the midst of the darkness they create, we may still find the light within that guides us on our way. Knowing that such light can be found and that through dealing with great sadness and almost impossible burdens we can glimpse, even faintly, that there is meaning in everything that happens in our lives, we can become not only stronger by taking on the challenges disease presents but we can feel ourselves transforming in greater and lesser ways. We can, shockingly, as Linda herself did, find the blessings in what life has brought us.

Linda shares her own journey in a readable and enjoyable way and by doing so offers real hope as well as good advice for those who find themselves in a similar situation. I am happy to recommend this book for any who are faced with disease either in themselves or in those they love.

~Dr. Jeffrey Raff
Jungian Analyst

Preface

Where the World Divides

To the parents,

Some way or another, all our worlds get divided. A family member may die abruptly, perhaps even violently (as in a car accident), or after a long deteriorating course. Someone you love suffers a major injury from which they won't fully recover. Your child is born with an illness or disability. Some big painful thing happens and your life gets split in two.

For us, that big painful thing is type 1 diabetes, which continues to rise on a global level each year. In my family, it happened twelve years ago when my son was two. For you, perhaps it is much newer. If so, it's likely you're in the search of your life. I'm sorry.

In writing this, I have tried to be cautious with your vulnerable state. I have tried not to give you too much. But even so, you may not be ready to hear all of the things you will read.

It's OK. If it becomes too much, go ahead and toss the book aside — throw it with some vigor against your closet door even. Let it fall to the floor and walk away. Never look at it again if you prefer. You don't have to force yourself to face all the realities right now.

Because right now, you have no idea what's coming up for you. You know nothing of how the rest of your life will go. If you're like I was, you don't know a thing about giving shots or what the insulin will do to blood sugar. You can't conceive now that you will gain power from the experience, and depending on how soon after diagnosis you're reading this, you might not care about the gold in illness, but I assure you it's right there among your deep and profound sadness. It's right in there with it, but you don't know. You're in shock at the moment, sticking needles in your child to save his life, trying to keep it all real as you do so. I'm sorry.

The entirety of this book was written with you in mind. May you find comfort in its words at this difficult time.

***

Normal levels of sugar in the bloodstream for someone with a healthy, working pancreas, as shown on a blood sugar meter, even immediately after consuming a large piece of cheesecake (I've checked):

70-100 mg/dl

Ty's range on any given day:

49-409 mg/dl

***

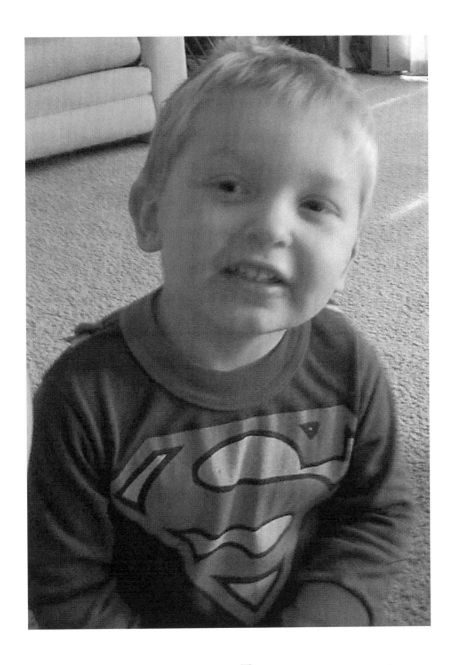

Ty

at the age of diagnosis

disease pain blame judgment lack of knowledge

frightened cry sadness every terror

pierce his finger and pinch my heart

swiftly shaken the heart is overcome with nervousness

driven Good mother protect child

Deeds done

With grief she turns away his my our hearts are sad

Chapter 1

Dreams

Dreams are the facts from which we must proceed.

~Carl Jung

I have studied dreams — my own and others — in my work in psychology for many years now, so it was not unusual for me to write down and reflect on the dream I had early in April 2000. In it, I took my diaper-clad son to a clinic, where a doctor told us "we" had diabetes. That was the end of the dream.

Realizing I knew nothing about diabetes, I looked it up in a medical book we had on the shelf to try to ascertain some symbolic meaning. I read about the symptoms and how the body tries to flush the excess sugar from itself, resulting in a constant thirst and heavy urination.

The Superman Years

Two weeks later my son's diapers, which had previously held an entire night's worth of urine, began to leak. I picked up the phone and hesitantly asked his pediatric nurse, "Is this anything?" She said probably not, but we should get a urine sample anyway. I'm sure you can see where this is going, but at the time I did not make the connection between my son's heavy diaper and the symptoms I had just read about two weeks before.

Yet you would think if a dream wanted to warn me about something this big, it would have spoken a little louder, maybe would have come to me in a little more booming way, or would have emitted a thunderbolt of emotion and caused me to wake in a cold sweat. It did not. The dream left me emotionally neutral. I woke easily from it. In fact, my only response was, "Oh. Ok." I was 100 percent accepting and alright with it. It was not so in waking life.

Dreams

Dream Come True

My husband, who is never out of town, was out of town. He had left Denver that morning to try to get to his grandfather in Ohio who wasn't doing well. A series of traveling obstacles (cancelled flights, weather), made it impossible for us to talk for more than a minute or two until ten thirty that night as he drove the last leg of his trip by rental car in the rain. By then, I'd known for five and a half hours.

I had scheduled a doctor's appointment for our son for that day, but neither one of us was very concerned. My son didn't appear sick, just cranky. I'd brought him in because I thought he was peeing excessively, and what's the worst that could be? He was two, and both symptoms could be chalked up to that.

So off Rob went on a plane and off I went with Ty and his three-year-old sister, Jalyn, to the doctor with a urine sample

I'd obtained by chasing him around the house with a bowl. After dropping the urine at the lab, I asked how long it would take, "Should I just wait here?"

"No, go ahead and take your kids home," the nurse said. "We'll call if the urine turns up anything but it's not likely." Five minutes later I pulled into our garage and my cell phone rang just as I had released and wrangled the kids out of their car seats. It was the doctor herself, telling us to come right back to the clinic. "Can it be anything else besides diabetes?" My words echoed as I spoke in the garage, "Can you tell me what it is?"

"Just come back and we'll talk about it," she told me.

So I wrangled and leashed two toddlers who had just gotten free back into their seats and we returned to the clinic.

I was never told the words, "Your son has diabetes." I think it would have helped to have heard it said concretely. Instead, a nurse gave an array of instructions I could not comprehend while I waited to hear what was wrong with my son.

Dreams

"Take this script to your pharmacy and get it filled. Then bring it back to us and we'll give him the shot here."

Confused, I asked, "What is it for?"

"Insulin," she said, her words slower and more compassionate, realizing her mistake.

"So he . . . does have diabetes," I said slowly, to give the words to myself. The nurse nodded.

I realize now the medical staff probably didn't know what to do with a positive diabetes test. They had to call and consult with a specialist on what to do and how to dose, as we were in "specialty" territory. They were likely scrambling for a plan to have in place for when I returned but got ahead of themselves and forgot about telling me what they knew . . . sugar in the urine, diabetes.

On the heels of this information, I left the clinic once again with toddlers in tow, back into their car seats to our pharmacy

25

wondering how I was expected to do this directly after *not* being told my son had diabetes. I held Ty on the counter while I rifled for the script.

"What's this for?" the pharmacist asked as I handed it to her.

"Um, insulin," and as I said the word, its meaning registered: I'm here getting this medicine my son needs to live and will forever need to live. As she walked away to fill it, I hid my head in the crook of Ty's neck and quietly cried.

Then back to the clinic we went, where a nurse drew up a syringe from the stuff I brought her and stuck it into my son's leg, followed by more incomprehensible instructions. I was to go to Barbara Davis first thing in the morning, the pediatrician said. I wondered, who was Barbara Davis . . . where did she live and why did I have to go to her house? They told me it was a diabetes specialty clinic in Denver we were very lucky to have so close by.

Dreams

Thank God I didn't know a thing about diabetes, knew no one who had it, and had no history of it in my family. My naivety saved me that first night. If I'd have known, there is no way I could have brought him home from the pediatrician's office on the instructions that if he seized in the night to call 911 (but they didn't expect his blood sugar to be down from 786 mg/dl by morning so I didn't have to worry).

***

Upon finally arriving home after this long day, I broke the news to family and friends, shed many tears, and voiced many fears; yet Rob still did not know about his son. Late that night in the dim and quiet of the nursery while my kids slept, we finally spoke. He was driving a rental car the last leg of his trip in a hard rain on a slick, rural Ohio road. I breathed deep and told it to him straight and level. Then I sat silent to receive his reaction. There was a long silence before he said, "So he does have this thing and he's going to have to deal with it for the rest of his life?"

"Yes."

He felt a well of panic as his body caught up to the news. All at once though, the rain stopped and simultaneously a distinct sense of peace, clarity, and calm encompassed him. With the sudden silence inside the darkness of the car, his attention was brought to the song playing on the radio—that hopeful, uplifting Johnny Nash song covered by Jimmy Cliff we all know, that goes,

I can see clearly now, the rain is gone
I can see all obstacles in my way
Gone are the dark clouds that had me blind
It's gonna be a bright (bright), bright (bright)
Sunshiny day

He told me it was like something was trying to tell him everything would be alright. It was a God moment, he said, and it was the first time I had ever heard him say such a thing.

Dreams

Things You Think You Cannot Do: Finger Pokes and Needles

Early the next morning, Ty and I went to the Barbara Davis Center, created by a mom whose daughter was diagnosed at a time when there was no specialty care. I felt better already. It seemed personal, like she had made it just for me. We made our way downtown and padded our way in our green fleece sleeper right up to the front desk.

His blood sugar, which they didn't expect to be down by morning, was 57, a very low number. They were cool about it, just gave him some juice, some graham crackers, and carried on—much different than my own reaction later that night when I dealt with my first low. The number 54 came up on the screen and I scrambled around like a madwoman, opening random cupboards looking for sugar before I got a handle on myself and told myself to be calm or else you'll scare the kids.

The Superman Years

I didn't know what the numbers meant yet—that I could easily have been met that night with a seizure. I'm glad I didn't know. In two days' time, I would know more than I ever wanted.

Out of all there was to break down about as I spent the long weekend at the clinic learning about the disease, it was the first finger poke that broke me open. I think I hid it. It's not good to stand over a two-year-old while wielding a needle and crying if you're trying to instill calm, so I hid it, but man did I feel the grief as I reached for my son's hand. It overwhelmed me, the sadness, perhaps because I knew this was the end of tender toddler fingertips. This first poke marked the beginning of all he would endure; the first invasion of the needle—the first of thousands. It was very hard for me to do. But of course, like we all must do, I did it.

"You'll be giving him his evening shot," the nurse educator said to me just as I was riding on the finger poke accomplishment.

"I will?" I asked, surprised. It hadn't occurred to me somehow. So foreign and anxiety-producing an action was this that I hadn't connected the necessity of the shots to me being the one giving them— not just this one time but tomorrow morning too, first thing. Shit.

"Ok," I said, trying to sound confident and willing. "No way in hell," I heard in my head, and made a mental note to wrangle out of it at some point over the next several hours.

Imperfect Insulin

Diabetes mellitus had been around since ancient times I was told. The Greeks called it a name meaning "sweet urine." He won't outgrow it, there is no cure, and he will be dependent on insulin every day for the rest of his life. Insulin is a hormone produced in the pancreas (a small organ behind the stomach), which opens cells to allow glucose from our food into them for nourishment. Without insulin, the glucose builds dangerously in the bloodstream.

It is a different disease than type 2 diabetes, where the pancreas may still produce insulin to varying degrees. In type 2, functioning can sometimes be improved with pills or by losing weight. In type 1, after the initial onset of symptoms, the pancreas will stop producing insulin altogether, making it necessary to inject it from the outside. No pills or diet will change that necessity.

There are two emergencies associated with the disease: ketosis (diabetic coma from high blood sugar), and insulin shock, caused by too much insulin which drops the amount of sugar in the bloodstream too low. The brain runs on sugar so, if deprived of glucose, it may cause the person to become disoriented, shaky, or sweaty. They may faint or lose consciousness and fall to the ground. My eyes widened at this and I remember thinking, *"This is the best you have for a disease that's been around since ancient times? All the medical miracles and this is the best that can be done for this one, a treatment that might kill the patient as much as save them?"* As soon as you learn this, the threat of seizure hangs over your head like a rigged axe and it is a huge burden.

"Oh yeah, and it's not a perfect science," the nurse continued. "We don't know what the right amount is. It changes every day." At least that's what I deduced from what she was saying.

No man-made thing works as elegantly as a healthy organ. The insulin we inject from the outside is grossly inefficient comparatively. But of course I gladly accepted it and immediately took my place among my ancestor diabetes mothers—the clan I had just become a part of. Thank God we had it. Insulin had only been made available for human use in the 1920s. Before that, one did not live with juvenile diabetes. Before that, my ancestors watched helplessly as their kids drifted into a high blood sugar coma and died. I was able to inject a resurrecting elixir into my son, watch him run, jump, play, laugh, and throw a ball. Not many parents of kids with chronic diseases or disabilities get to do that.

Later I met with a mental health therapist who dealt with psychological issues specific to this disease. She told me Ty didn't get diabetes because of anything I did or fed him or because he had too much sugar, and this helped immensely as I was ruing the hotdogs I'd allowed him to eat and the giant sweet tarts I craved while pregnant with him.

She asked me if I knew anyone with diabetes. No I did not. She asked, "What's the image that forms in your mind when you think of someone with diabetes?" She was trying to dispel any myths or misinformation I might hold. I pictured an overweight person, but that's as specific as I could get. I didn't even know the connection. I realized I had no idea. What would someone with diabetes look like? Would they look ill, or overweight, or walk with a limp?

My husband is a Rehabilitation Psychologist. He works with people with disabilities. What he knew about diabetes at diagnosis he saw daily in his clients—blindness, kidney failure, end-stage disability. This was the image of my son's future which formed immediately in his mind when he heard the news, he told me later. I had it better for my ignorance.

As I tried to formulate my answer, I heard laughter at the front desk outside the glass windows of the playroom where we were training. I looked up to see a family—a mother, a father, and a little girl about Ty's age. The nurse said they were Craig and Nancy Crease, and little Emily Crease, known well around the center because Craig, who also sells insulin pumps to the clinic, has type 1 and so did their little girl, who was only a year older than Ty. Emily had already had the disease for two years.

I looked at them standing there laughing—they were laughing! I thought, "Oh, so this is what someone with diabetes looks like—happy, healthy, and cute." I took a deep breath, so greatly relieved, and continued with the day in a way I would not have been able to had they not been standing there.

We are not sure how we subsequently met and discovered we lived close to one another, but the Creases have been great friends to us all these years. I just attended Craig's fiftieth birthday party, laughed a lot, and once again left feeling so uplifted by being understood. Nancy and I share so many common concerns, there is just nothing like it.

***

"Couldn't you give him the shot before we leave the clinic today?" I snuck that in randomly while the nurse educator was talking about something else. "I'll feed him dinner right when I get home." The negotiations had begun.

"You'll be ready to do it by then, you will," she tried to assure me. I nodded my head not believing her one bit.

She told me if I really, really didn't want do it that night, she wouldn't make me. Immediately in my head I heard, "Yes, yes, I'll take that option. I really, really don't want to do it tonight."

"But if you don't do it tonight," she continued, "you will only worry about it all night and create that much more dread around it."

I'm willing to risk it, I thought. But I understood she was right. Sooner or later I was going to have to suck it up and do it.

"Alright, I'll give him his evening shot," I conceded, and could take in no other instructions that afternoon for the distraction of this thought.

Perhaps she would have liked to have gone home after a long day of trying to teach crucial, life-saving techniques to distraught parents. In the end, however, our nurse, Cindy, taking pity on me in my husband's absence, graciously and angelically came to my house after we left the clinic that day to support me through the first solo shot. She stood by me in the kitchen and taught me to draw up the insulin outside of Ty's line of sight, to deal with my fear before approaching him with the needle, and to move calmly but quickly as I administered the shot into his thigh. She sat down with me on the playroom floor where I held Ty in my lap and spoke close to my shoulder, coaching and encouraging. I did it just as she instructed.

Ty looked up at me funny as if to see if he should be OK with what I just did. I smiled and kissed him on the cheek, squeezed his shoulder, and told him, "Good job." Then Cindy had me get up and let Ty get on with his playing. Minimize the drama, she advised, don't make it into some big emotional thing.

While taking a breath out after the first shot, it occurred to me that I would have to face a finger poke again soon. This time, there would be no nurse by my shoulder—no back up—just me, alone in my house with my two toddlers.

That night, I retreated to the kids' bathroom to prepare myself. I didn't want to do it. I sat on top of the toilet seat half crying, shaking my head in one hand, holding the meter, strips, and lancet in the other. I made my resolve and collected myself. When I looked up, Ty was standing right in front of me, still in his green sleeper, with his index finger held up in the air, making it easier for me.

***

In the dead of night, after a borderline blood sugar check I was not sure how to handle, I called my sister. She is a registered nurse in Minneapolis and triages after-hours urgent calls. I felt so lost, not knowing the behavior of the monster. As she explained things to me in the middle of the night, I thought, "She is the one equipped to deal with this, not me." I deal with the psyche, not the body.

The Superman Years

Not every nurse would have known as much as she did about the disease. As I listened to her in the darkness, she told me she thought it weird, given Ty's diagnosis, that she had a special interest in diabetes in nursing school. She found diabetes really interesting when most students did not, she said. It was too complicated and hard to learn for them and required too much specialized knowledge.

When my friend Craig (diabetic since age seven), met with his surgeon regarding a shoulder surgery, the doctor asked if his pump needed to be connected during surgery! We are the specialists now. We know what many non-specialists don't know, that insulin-dependent means you need to be hooked up to it or you die. The fact that someone who's going to be operating on you doesn't know this could strike the fear of God into you, but diabetes is its own entity, a wildly complex and shifty beast one really can't "get" in medical school unless it's your specialty. Craig's wife was there to make sure his blood sugar was managed properly while he was under.

Dreams

I walked into the clinic early the next morning, two toddlers in tow, feeling much lighter for another eight hour day of education and training. The morning shot had been far easier on my psyche and Rob was scheduled to come home later that afternoon.

The staff asked if I wouldn't mind joining another "new onset" family for an educational session with the endocrinologist. "Sure," I agreed. I walked into the consultation room with Jalyn and Ty, joking and laughing a bit with the staff, but was immediately met with a wave of heaviness that stopped me in my tracks. Looking back at me were the horribly stricken faces of a mother and father with their nine-year-old son. He had just been released from the hospital after nearly falling into a coma at the time of his diagnosis. Their news was one day newer than mine and I realized, with a little shock, that that very well may have been what my face looked like just a day before.

The Superman Years

Their son was named Tyler also, and this created a certain kinship among us. They were emotionally fragile and tearful on and off throughout the teaching session. When the doctor stepped out of the room for something, the father pointed to a folder of information the clinic provides for new families. "Did you read the yellow sheet in here?" he asked, incredulous. I replied I had not. I had somehow not even seen that one. "Good!" he said shaking his head tearfully, "Don't read it." The doctor walked back in the room just then and I wondered for the rest of the day what terrible thing could be on that sheet of paper. Weren't seizures and comas the worst of it?

We drove straight to the airport after leaving the clinic late that afternoon to pick up Rob. He stepped into the car and started joking around with the kids, making us all happy like everything would be OK.

It was nice to hear Jalyn giggle. In some ways I felt worse for her than I did for Ty. A quiet, shy, and sweet child, it was Jalyn who seemed traumatized by the whole thing. The sight of the needles going into her brother really frightened her and when they had to draw her blood that day to see if she might be at risk for diabetes also, she struggled and cried. Even months later when we went to the dentist, I told him, "Too soon for needles for this one." She remembers more of Ty's diagnosis than he does.

By the time we arrived at our house, it was time for the next shot. I slowly gave Rob meticulous and overly detailed instructions on dosing, drawing up, and injecting the insulin. But before I finished demonstrating on my own leg how to hold the skin, how to punch the needle through quickly but plunge the insulin in slowly to avoid a sting, Rob walked over to Ty and simply gave him the shot, like it was no big deal.

I walked by Ty's room upstairs and noticed its condition. You couldn't see the floor. How did it get so trashed when we hadn't even been home for the better part of three days? But toddlers cover a lot of ground in a short amount of time, and trashed it was with toys, empty juice boxes and straw wrappers, and books and papers strewn in all directions. Instinctively, I walked in and started picking up a few things, then despite myself, kneeled down in it and started sorting piles. Over by the closet was the folder from the clinic. It was open and empty. Under a pile of toys were the brochures. There was the yellow sheet, the one the father told me not to read, upside down and stuck to a purple sheet by a mysterious substance, thereby mercifully saving my psyche until now. I slowly reached for it against my better judgment, pulled the papers apart, and started to read. It was titled, "Complications of Type 1 Diabetes." It was a good thing I was on my knees already.

Truthfully, I'm not even going to lay them out for you here in case you have been spared thus far. I don't want you to hear it from me. I cannot, even now, get through the list when someone asks about the long-term effects of high blood sugar and what can happen over time.

Dreams

As I absorbed the final sad fact, Rob poked his head in to ask a question, registered the look on my face and asked, "What's wrong?" I shook my head. "I just read this thing I wasn't supposed to read." I knew I was about to cry, but sick of all the intermittent crying I had been doing all weekend, I tried to rush past Rob in the doorway to spare him the intensity. Things had been so much more upbeat today and I didn't want to ruin it with more devastating realizations. "Linda," he caught my arm and pulled me back to him. "I know, I feel it too," and I could see that he did, just as much as me. We had our first joint cry there embraced in the doorway. What a different experience than crying alone.

Another long night loomed ahead, but we were all together now. At the kids' bedtime we dimmed the lights of the nursery, crawled around Ty in his bed and pressed play just like we did every night. Ty pointed to the screen and said, "La la" (his name for the future Lion King, Simba, which was having a nightly run at our house for the past, oh, year or so). As the triumphant, celebratory *Circle of Life* theme began, with the darkness like a cocoon around us, I felt enormously comforted by the simple ritual. Even with all the momentous changes of the last few days, at least this part of our lives was intact—that come bedtime, we were all home, safe and secure together. Not everyone has that luxury in the days following diagnosis.

dark black
nights
and days

this
daze

trance travelers
within the self
go-between distant lands

the light of stars
well hidden in thick DARKNESS

yet,
indeed,
heaven is wrapped in darkness

Chapter 2

Coma

My friend, Barb, didn't have the option of taking her one-year-old daughter, Jacqueline, home the day she was diagnosed; and her husband was a lot farther away than Ohio. He was in Malaysia, and she was taking care of her mother who was dying.

I said I would be careful with your vulnerability, and already I'm talking about one of the most frightening experiences associated with this disease. Yet this is the way many kids are diagnosed with type 1 diabetes, after it has become an emergency situation involving the brain. Many are forced to face this harsh reality at the outset.

The Superman Years

Barb had taken her baby to the doctor several weeks prior, on her mother's suggestion, after her mother had noticed some weight loss in Jacqueline. After a cursory check of her ears, nose, and throat, this doctor lectured Barb on being an over-reactive first-time mother. She felt embarrassed that she had wasted his time.

One month later, Barb watched as Jacqueline lay listless and semi-conscious on an emergency room table, breathing a shallow loud breath Barb told me you would never forget if you heard. Then the ER staff whisked her away for immediate medical attention and Barb braced herself to make the phone call to her husband ten thousand miles away. She had to explain to him that their daughter's brain was swelling and that there was only a 50 percent chance they would get her back.

Jacqueline spent the next three days unconscious in ICU while they worked to stabilize her blood sugar and reduce the brain swelling. Barb recalls, it was on the third night that

Coma

Jacqueline woke in a screaming cry. The doctors said she likely had a nasty headache from the brain swelling and the still-high blood sugar. She cried the rest of the time at the hospital—two more days—while Barb learned all about drawing up and injecting insulin, balancing carbohydrates, etc. Unable to face the flight back to Malaysia where they were living, her husband, Terry, cut short his contract and returned to the United States.

Coma is a deeply mysterious, little understood state of consciousness from which the person cannot be woken from outside stimuli. Traditionally, in the medical world, communication with the person in coma has been attempted from the outside through shakes of the shoulders, jabs, and pokes. But one Jungian analyst I know attempts communication on a different level. Dr. Arnold Mindell is a doctor who conducts psychotherapy with people in coma.

Dr. Mindell uses a unique approach. He figures out a way to communicate with those in coma by mimicking any kind of vocalizations, body twitches, or movements the person may make. So, for instance, if an eye twitched, Dr. Mindell would place a finger near the eye and twitch it again in the same manner. Soon a yes/no system is established, like one eye twitch for yes and two for no, or something similar. A different person in a coma might be able to communicate with a toe movement for example.

One of the most intriguing stories he recounts in his book, *Coma: The Dreambody Near Death* (2009), is about a guy he calls "Sam," who had been stuck in coma for six months. Sam made a number of loud guttural and vocal noises, whoops, and hoots. The hospital staff had actually come to see him as a bit of an annoyance, as you can imagine loud noise would only add to their already stressful work.

Dr. Mindell was able to establish communication by exaggerating these vocals; so if Sam would go, "Whoooooo," Dr. Mindell would repeat it louder and with exaggeration, no doubt causing the staff, other patients, and visitors to wonder about his credibility. After some back and forth of this, the loud "whoooo" turned into a "WOW"! Dr. Mindell asked Sam about what he was seeing and why he was saying "wow." Sam became lucid enough to start talking right then, and said he saw a white ship—common imagery (white vessels of some sort) in dreams of people who are near death.

Dr. Mindell guided Sam as if through a dream. He encouraged Sam to go check out the ship, to see where it was going, and to decide if he wanted to take that ship. Sam did so, and found that it was going to Bermuda. He wondered if he could take that ship being that he had a job that he needed to go to everyday. Could he really take that vacation?

At this point, Dr. Mindell had to step out of the room for a short time and told Sam to contemplate that question. Sam fell into a deep restful state—sort of half snoring. A few minutes later, Dr. Mindell returned. Sam apparently decided to take the ship to Bermuda after all. He had quietly passed.

Clearly there is more going on in our inner, psychological world and in altered states of consciousness than most realize, whether any part of the experience is remembered or not. Dr. Mindell believes some deeply important psycho spiritual process is being worked out for the person. Perhaps it is our job to trust that we, and the doctors, are not the only ones caring for coma patients while they are in their vastly altered states.

Being one year old at the time, Jacqueline remembers nothing of her experience (although I'm sure her parents will never forget), but maybe your child does. You should ask. Do they recall any part of going in or coming out of the coma? Did they experience anything like a dream, or do they remember vivid body sensations like floating or crashing through space?

People coming out of coma commonly talk of stars and space. The experience ultimately alters their life direction (with or without memory during coma), and sets them on a specific course, even if they were in a coma as a child. Perhaps something about the mysterious experience is significant for their future and may forge certain characteristics into their personalities that will ultimately benefit those around them.

I'm happy to tell you that Jacqueline is something like six feet tall now and soon off to college. She has lived in Malaysia, speaks fluent Mandarin, plays the violin, and is a great golfer. She and her parents are quite the survivors, just like many of you.

wounded

lost

hurt

the tender conversation

the sidelong glances

turning her whole
attention
to an angry
beast

Though
they
turn
away
in
tears
hearts
are
joined

confronting it
a young son's
body
teaches

does
she
hope
to win?

my child
he has courage
The Hero

Chapter 3

Powerlessness

It was easy to love God in all that was beautiful. The lessons of deeper knowledge, though, instructed me to embrace God in all things.

~St. Francis of Assisi

Don't Demand Perfection Unless You Like to Fail Repeatedly and For the Rest of Your Life

After the medical visits taper down from the initial marathon sessions to once every few months, in a short time you go from helpful, knowledgeable, and understanding medical staff to a world where no one else seems to have diabetes or understand it. Daily life with the disease begins and you kind of look around your house with a bewildered feeling knowing nothing is the same. The experience changes from, "What will this be like?" to "Here is what it is."

If cluelessness saved me that first night, it was pure adrenaline that got me through the next few months. I felt in a constant state of nervous system activity—my brain and body emitting a "tired but wired" kind of feeling. There seemed no time to think about anything else but getting this down, getting this right, never making a mistake, and controlling blood sugar.

My personal quest was to get a number "in-range" every time we tested Ty's blood sugar. Anyone see a problem with this? We checked his blood sugar about every two hours, sometimes more, and charted every number, trying to control for all the variables. I peered into them, looking again and again to see if any patterns emerged; searching for a magic combination of insulin dose and number of carbohydrates which would produce the same results twice, but this has still yet to happen. Too many factors affect blood sugar: foods, insulin, exercise, growth hormones, even a change in season for God's sake. It's impossible to predict which factor is going to affect blood sugar in which direction and when.

With all these variables, the insulin does not perform reliably. Sometimes it absorbs rapidly and overshoots the mark and sometimes it doesn't seem to work at all—an hour and a half later, the same or an even higher number appears on the meter screen. It doesn't take long to realize insulin dosing is really no more than a "guess, hope, and pray" kind of decision every time. You inject the insulin and hope it works right this time. Pray I don't drop him to the floor.

With exercise, one of two things might happen: the amount of sugar in the bloodstream might go high or it might go low. Physical exertion generally drops blood sugar very quickly; however, if there's not enough insulin in the bloodstream to open the cells to sugar, or if stored sugar in the muscles and the liver is released in response to adrenaline, then it will go high for awhile before it is settles back into the muscles and drops sugar unexpectedly hours later, perhaps deep in the night. If you are one who likes things concrete and predictable when it comes to keeping your child safe, you may silently begin to go crazy about now.

For months I kept learning some new thing about the disease I didn't know before, usually the hard way. One time early on I checked Ty after a bath and caught him at a low number at which he should not have been able to stand. After I treated it, I called the clinic in a panic. Oh yeah, they said, if you give him a warm bath too soon after a shot, it will open the capillaries and allow the insulin to be absorbed too quickly and cause a bad low.

We also didn't know, even living in the Rocky Mountains, that a change in altitude affects blood sugar. When we thought we were settling into the life a bit, we decided to try to be a normal family and do what we would normally do — go to the mountains for a weekend, rent a boat, and spend some time on the lake. It would be good for us, we thought, to maybe breathe a little again.

We had so many blood sugar readings in the three hundreds that all we wanted to do was come back down the mountain to our house where we had had better luck. (That was also the same weekend we accidentally drowned the meter in the bait box without having brought a back up. We were such rookies. You never do that more than once).

Consumed as I was with the learning curve, I had not even considered what Ty might deal with as an adult until I caught wind of a conversation between two fishermen casting just offshore early one morning on a glassy Wisconsin lake where my husband and I both grew up. I had taken my coffee to sit on the docked pontoon in the dappled morning sunlight and it was the first time I had felt relaxed in a long while. Sounds carry from great distances with great clarity over water and I could hear them perfectly. I tuned in when one was telling the other a story about a buddy of his who was arrested just the other night, put down on the ground, and handcuffed. I listened to hear what his buddy had done. In the north woods of Wisconsin, it could be any number of entertaining, drunken reasons.

"Turns out it was his blood sugar." *You've got to be kidding*, I thought to myself. He explained the guy was having a low and resembled an agitated drunk person. He was unable to respond to the officer's orders.

Ty was so young when I heard this I didn't picture him yet as a man possibly in need of emergency medical attention in the future, and that he might be shoved to the ground and shackled for it. I shook my head and headed up to the cabin, peacetime over. There would be a long road of challenges ahead that I could not even imagine.

As Above, So Below

I handle hard things well, I always have. Years of crisis work in psychiatric hospitals honed an ability to keep calm in highly tense situations. I was determined to handle all of this the same way, but it turns out I was a bit grandiose in my vision. After just a few months of trying to juggle all the variables, the adrenaline seemed to fizzle out all at once and a sadness hit me the likes of which I had never known.

Funny how your psyche protects itself and gives you what you can take in pieces. Three months of knowing what the disease was all about—living it—and I still had not made the connection that it was never going away. I was doing nothing more than walking down the basement stairs for yet another blood sugar check when the full realization of the word "chronic" hit me so unexpectedly and deeply that my knees buckled a little. It is one thing to intellectually understand a thing and another to experience it when it hits the level of the body. I had just gotten it.

The realization ushered in a period of deep struggle. How would I ever be able to keep this up? I felt weak and tired already and it was just the start. It reminded me of childbirth when they told me the hard labor had not even begun when I was 1 cm dilated after eight hours and the gal in the next room was 8 cm after one hour. There was just no way I could take it. Then a book passed in front of my face called, *Anatomy of the Spirit*, by Carolyn Myss, that gave me the correct perspective at this critical juncture when I was in despair.

She reminded me that everything we do in the physical world is at once symbolic. Like the Hermetic phrase, "as above, so below," everything has a higher and a lower meaning. So when you take a shower you cleanse your physical body and your physical hair. But as the water flows over your scalp, there is a psychic cleansing as well. When you step out of the shower, you feel cleaner, psychically lighter, relieved of something. When you clean out a cluttered drawer, there is a similar effect in your mind. When you put your hands in prayer position, a reverent feeling is invoked just by the physical action, even before you begin to pray. So too, do the origins of disease lie in the heavens, inseparable from the physical.

Holding this perspective through great difficulty gave me a way to see the bigger story going on beyond the pancreas. To cope, I would have to gather all of it in my acceptance (the good, the bad, and the extremely difficult), and accept it all as divinely gifted.

It changes everything, because now you see your work as a sacred charge. It doesn't mean it won't be hard, grueling, and exhausting, but it will have purpose. You will happily do it because you have been entrusted to it. You must be the exact right person to do this. You *are* doing it. You diligently learn all the necessary care routines, give the injections, check blood sugar readings religiously, and plan for all contingencies. Of course you're the one to do it.

Professional Changes

I quit my job after diagnosis. At the time, I was working as a therapist in psychiatric hospitals, the kind where the doors lock with a loud clang behind you. It involved long hours in a high-stress, intense, crisis environment. I loved it for a long time. I learned a ton, and what I saw in the individuals who stayed there bore great compassion in me.

But after diagnosis there was no way I could keep up the rigors of hospital work. Actually, I couldn't keep up with them before. It was one thing when I was young and single, but trying to relax and pump breast milk for a half-hour once in a twelve-hour crisis hospital shift started not working for me.

But I guess it provided some measure of safety and comfort in my skills because I wouldn't leave. I hung in there much past knowing it was no longer for me—through pregnancies and births—resenting the environment versus exercising my freewill to leave. I'd work twelve-hour shifts eight-months pregnant, and sometimes go to the emergency room for a psychiatric assessment in the middle of the night after that. There were lots of stress hormones circulating constantly, and don't think I haven't thought about those conditions having something to do with the situation we have now.

Diagnosis helped me quit. Given the consuming nature of the learning curve and the daily care involved with diabetes, I was truly not even thinking or caring about my professional future. The real psychological work was happening right here in my life, I knew, in the experience of the disease.

But one starry Colorado night on my deck, I saw myself teaching in front of a classroom. The image infused me with energy and in a flash of insight, I knew I was seeing my future. Having no experience or connections in this area though, I wondered how I would ever break in to teaching. It seemed very far away and inaccessible in the stars.

One misdirected inquiry call later, to the "wrong" professor at a local college, and an easy, casual conversation about education and work history led to an appointment as a psychology professor for the past eleven years, which has been a great gig for me. The trajectory of my work changed in a way for which I am forever grateful.

***

If I needed you, Would you come to me? Would you come to me and ease my pain?

If you needed me, I would come to you, I would swim the seas for to ease your pain.

You will miss sunrise, if you close your eyes, and that would break my heart in two.

~Lyle Lovett

Powerlessness

Don't ask me how, don't ask me when, but I think we were pretty far into the first year before Rob and I got away for a night. Besides being scared to leave, we had no family around, nor did we have a babysitter. It's not like you're going to teach the fifteen-year-old down the street how to give shots quick so you can go out. It was Katy, a college student with type 1 herself who we met at the clinic that gave us enough confidence and peace of mind to venture out for one night. We only had her a short, blessed time before she moved on to nursing school so she could work directly with the hospitalized kids with diabetes. Kind of selfish of her to leave us in the lurch like that.

We went to an outdoor concert at Red Rocks Amphitheatre just up the road from our house. If you're not familiar, it is one of the coolest, most naturally beautiful places to see live music in the country. An amphitheater of giant red rock outcroppings in the foothills above Denver. The steep rock walls form an arc of natural acoustics. Shakespeare plays were performed here before the days of sound systems. As the sun sets behind you, the entire surround glows in orange and red. As dusk darkens the bright blue Colorado skies, the sprawling lights of Denver shimmer across the valley below. Silently taking in this beautiful scene together that first night away from our duties, Rob started to say something but his voice caught and he stopped — he shook his head and looked away. I saw that he was tearful. I knew it had to do with Ty and a lump formed in my throat before he spoke. I waited for him to continue.

He gestured toward the peak of one of the giant rocks glowing in the sunset, "Do you ever worry that Ty might not be able to see this someday?" My chest lurched before he got the words out and I waited before I responded.

"You worry about his eyes?" I asked, this being previously undisclosed information. "I don't know," I paused. "I worry about his kidneys."

Powerlessness

We cried for the rest of the night, each in turn moved by the music and the beauty. He tried to hide it from me and I tried to hide it from him, but we both knew.

I know this does not sound like a great first night out, but actually, it was just what we needed. When you're at home on the front lines you're running around, focused on insulin to carbohydrate ratios and the six thousand other factors affecting blood sugar levels, while working around the clock to prevent seizures. There's not a lot of "down time" to reflect on deeper meanings and bigger pictures. It connected us, experiencing the sadness and the worn-outedness together in a beautiful place with beautiful music. Beautiful guitar combined with beautiful piano. Difficult emotion and beauty existed side-by-side, sacred with the profane, so exquisitely mixed. I was glad for the feeling of solidarity—we were in this together—and I was grateful because years later, the cumulative effect of these same forces would pull us apart down to the last thread.

Cure Parties: To Dream or Not to Dream; Idealism vs. Reality

The first time I attended a Juvenile Diabetes Research Foundation fundraiser (on the invitation of another mother who happened to be in the pediatric clinic the day of diagnosis), it had only been a couple of months since diagnosis so I was very emotional. I took every bid personally, holding myself back from going up to everyone saying, "Thank you, thank you," emphatically with my hands clasped to my heart. Just one of those drinks (the way they make them at those things), and a new diagnosis is not a good mix.

The next year I attended, I spoke. I delivered a speech. Now, I have no natural inclination to put myself in front of a couple hundred people and a spotlight, yet this is exactly what I found myself actually asking to do. I wrote an impassioned speech, practiced it a million times, and still wanted to throw up in the days and hours leading up to it.

Powerlessness

Despite another year and a couple of months since diagnosis, I was still very emotional. I spoke of my love/hate relationship with insulin, of that intimidating red glucagon kit which forever sits in our armoire, the constant threat of seizure, and the lost innocence of an ice cream cone at the pool. But in closing I offered an image of a different potential future I saw for our kids—one in which a large group of us are celebrating by a huge bonfire, saying a few words of gratitude over our no-longer-needed lancets, needles, and insulin vials, before throwing them all up into the fire.

It was probably too much. I'm not sure everyone there wanted to hear the raw emotion of a parent. But looking out over the crowd as the lights came up, I saw plenty of faces with glistening eyes who got it, plenty personally involved with the disease. When I returned to my table after the speech there was a woman—a mother—waiting by my chair to talk to me, crying. Her daughter had been diagnosed years before but she related to so much I had said. My husband sat silenced, which believe me never happens.

What I remember most about that speech is how much I knew the image could be true. It wasn't like wishful thinking or the deluded fantasy of a desperate parent, but more like solid knowledge of the possibility.

Years ago I sent out an inquiry to parents on a major diabetes website for something I was writing at the time. I asked them how they envisioned celebrating the cure. I had expected to receive all kinds of great, celebratory visions. Instead, the responses were, "I haven't really thought about it," or "I have to live as if there will never be a cure," and even, "the cure is not discussed at our house." They were quick to point out though, that this didn't mean they didn't want a cure more than anything else.

I was a bit taken back, but then I looked at how far out of diagnosis they were. These were the long-timers, most ten to eighteen years out.

Powerlessness

I've been at it twelve years so I understand their responses much better now. We have suffered setbacks and painful disappointments regarding advancements and a cure, yet we must continue with the regimen just like we've been doing year after year, day after day. I understand the parents' stance. We'll keep doing what we need to do. Call us when there's a cure.

It's a painful place to live in hope; "unrealistic," one parent called it. Painful, I think because most of us know a cure actually exists out there in the ether, and if only we could catalyze it, we could stop our kids' complications in their tracks. They could run and play free of the apparatus needed to keep them alive. It is hard to hold hope when the disease continues to march on in the body and we feel powerless to stop it.

I know when I am strong in the feeling though, it is like an energy with tangible power. It is something that carries me through the routine, lifts me up, and helps me endure. I wondered after I read the parents' responses, would I, too, lose this hope I was riding on? The answer was "yes," but I didn't

expect to feel it leave me so abruptly.

Deeply from within my heart
a dwelling place for suffering

wet-eyed
despairing
cracked
choked with grief

am I
strong enough
to bear its
wrath

A heart
undone

no
sleep
could defeat
me.

sacred
yoga meditation breath
that which leads us to peace

Chapter 4

Sleep Deprivation

Very likely because of my son's particular illness, and because I had a diagnosis dream send me down a particular path in my research and teaching, I became immersed and wildly interested in the whole world of altered consciousness, dreams, and shamanism. Whereas a doctor you know may bring medical training and skills to treat a patient, a shaman (part priest, therapist, doctor, midwife, and ritual maker to a community), brings the healing into another realm — the one just above our heads.

Shamans' work happens in an altered state of consciousness, achieved by dreaming, drumming, chanting, praying, meditating, ingesting hallucinogenic plants, fasting, or severely depriving themselves of sleep. In such states, one can "travel."

The Superman Years

The way most of us have experienced this ability to be somewhere else is in a dream. One is not bound by the laws of physics or knowledge available only in the physical plane. In dream-like visions, a shaman might diagnose an illness, receive directions for treating the patient, or find the location of a plant which bears the correct medicine.

What I find so interesting about dreams is that we all have them. In all times, in all cultures, every human dreams. It binds us globally at this moment to all other humans, as well as to our ancestors throughout the ages.

Some of the prominent theories of dreams is that they are random neuronal firing during sleep, but I know this is terribly reductionist. Yes, your brain is bursting with activity during a dream, but dreams are much more than that.

To many, the usefulness of dreams is too far out of the box to spend time paying attention to them. But those drawn into them know they are an access point into a great mystery—a world much different than our day to day. Dreams take us way down into the primal part of ourselves where we remember ritual and meditation and prayer, past the worry and concern where we know it is true. And we all have them, as above so below, there is divine in man.

A shaman is called into their work by a dream, and have often spent their childhoods in initiation, "travelling between the realms" of consciousness, usually due to debilitating childhood illnesses or disabilities which caused them fever, delirium, seizure, to have a near-death experience, coma, or oxygen-deprivation (as with asthma). It is as if they have had a lot of practice altering consciousness. Eventually though, the individual overcomes the physical and psychological obstacles they have faced and bring their new strengths and powers back to the benefit of the community — the classic hero's journey.

The Superman Years/The Bush Years

It started out with the Superman pajamas, the kind with the Velcro red cape. Ty spotted them, put them on ironically just before diagnosis, and they didn't seem to come off for a few years. He wore them day and night, outside and inside. We painted his room classic red and royal blue and added Superman bedding and accessories. Several birthday parties in a row were Superman-themed with Superman cake.

He upgraded his everyday Superman look with deluxe Superman costumes on several Halloweens: one with a fan inside that inflated phony muscles, another with a flashing light that circled the diamond-shaped "S" emblem on his chest, and one with built-in abs, pectorals, and biceps. All the grandparents, aunts and uncles, and friends fully supported his alter ego by giving him Superman gifts on all occasions. We had Superman swim trunks and Superman backpacks, a Superman

84

nightlight, and a Superman lamp. But you're not allowed to blatantly show your superhero nature much past first grade, so during the transition to appearing merely mortal, he lost the cape and graduated to superman T-shirts, sweatshirts, and baseball caps in every variety.

The Superman theme from the Christopher Reeve movies resounded through my house at all times of the day, accompanying all our daily tasks. I could not think of a more apt archetype to carry him through this disease—diabetes his only kryptonite. Every hero has a weak spot.

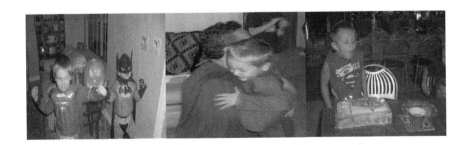

Superhero Incarnate

What Ty didn't realize as he flew around the house, the cul-de-sac, and Target, with arms and fists straight out in front of him, was that the guy on the screen was my hero too. Ty was diagnosed during an era of good hope. Stem cell research was all the talk and showed the most promise for a cure. It seemed all the factors were lined up for it to actually happen! Scientists were working diligently in the lab, excited about this avenue of research. Doctors (octogenarians who had devoted their lives to treating patients and advancing research), were more than ready to see this milestone in their lifetimes — to see their work come to fruition. Many who suffered the diseases and disability which stood to be done away with by this research, like Multiple Sclerosis, some forms of cancer, spinal cord injuries, and Parkinson's, were standing up, raising awareness, and advocating (including Ty's grandmother, paralyzed many years before, who served on the National JDRF board and flew to Washington more on behalf of Ty than herself). We had a potential opportunity to witness an amazing miracle in our lifetime, so many illnesses cured! I could imagine it and I could feel the happy magnitude of it.

Christopher Reeve, despite his catastrophic injury, became a powerful voice for our family as he advocated stem cell research. It was an ironic, happy coincidence to me—big Superman helping little Superman. I don't think it gets more potent than Superman in a wheelchair, rising up on behalf of others. I felt a part of something revolutionary, even though all I could do was watch from the sidelines, clap and cheer, and be grateful to those speaking for me and influencing in a way I could not. He didn't have to do this with his injury and no one would have blamed him if he didn't. I'm sure it was exhausting and dangerous for him to travel and speak with the heft of his required medical needs.

I could tell though, that he knew in the same way I did that so much suffering was wholly unnecessary. I longed to ask him the same question I asked those parents on the website because I knew without a doubt that he had a clear plan for the celebration he would literally walk into. Then, bam, all that hope and promise and potential came to a screeching halt.

I watched from the edge of my seat, hands over my mouth, as former president George W. Bush halted government funding of stem cell research. That was the moment. I felt a literal drain—a deflation—hope directly leaving me. I knew with that announcement, Ty's chances were set back many years, and that we had probably lost our window for his lifetime. I couldn't believe it. I naively assumed everyone wanted a cure for diseases and disability. How did my son's potential cure become such a huge political entanglement?

Of course not everyone who opposed understood the research, and their position was often based less on strongly cherished beliefs than false assumptions regarding the science which was fairly new at the time. It came down to unawareness and a lack of education (not in all cases, but in many). This came easier for those of us whose health depended on it. We educated ourselves, knew the cells were harvested from those in excess stored in infertility clinics being otherwise thrown in the garbage to the tune of 400,000/year. We knew there was no intent for human cloning (as some assumed and feared). We knew that the potential in these embryos was in the many lives they could save, not in the garbage where they were ending up.

Sometime after his announcement, Bush appeared on TV with several couples standing behind him with their "snowflake babies" — babies adopted as frozen embryos from in-vitro fertility clinics. My mouth hung open. Truly was this what he was proposing as the solution? For the country to thaw out and adopt 400,000 embryos each year? Despite the heroics of Mr. Reeve, the president used his first two vetoes to keep the decision from being overturned.

89

After that, everything got very quiet. I didn't do well psychologically. The decision put a whole new spin on Ty's diabetes. It made the sleep deprivation and daily care overwhelming. I was exhausted. Rob was exhausted. We were sick with grief and powerlessness. I felt alone again, back in the trenches of the daily care, toiling away.

Silent Consequences

I've never read an account of the method a shaman might use to deprive her or himself of sleep, usually by waking themselves repeatedly. The method I unwittingly adopted was worrying over an illness that required constant monitoring and setting an alarm clock to go off every couple hours for twelve years. It has been pretty effective.

To give you an idea, let me tell you about last night. Although particularly brutal, it happens often enough. Ty had eaten pizza at a friend's house, thereby wrecking his blood

90

sugar and my sleep. The check before bed was fine, but as I predicted, two hours later it was sky high. Two hours after that, it was as if I had not given him any insulin—still really high. Now the worry that he will start to get sick from such high blood sugar joins in. Two hours after that, down about one hundred points, still high though. By dawn, we had turned the corner, but only after nine hours and some unusually high doses of insulin.

A more typical night consists of two or three checks; maybe half the time he needs some insulin, or maybe some juice. These are the nights I have come to hope for.

I certainly do not want to scare you into thinking my fate is definitely yours. I know plenty of type 1 diabetes parents who do not live like this (it's not everyone's lot), but I also know plenty who do. Our son's blood sugar just happens to get more volatile at night. There's no logical reason for it of course. We have caught him at dangerous numbers often enough to warrant checks every night. People have a hard time believing we get up as often as we do.

I've come to believe unrelenting sleep loss is one of the most neglected and serious side effects of this disease, and you may need a plan in place to care for yourself. Along with grief, it has been one of the hardest aspects for me to deal with personally. And when the two occur together (which they usually do), well, you have yourself a powerful mix.

Your doctors are not going to tell you to get up every two hours in the night and check blood sugar. They know how harmful this would be. The clinic staff will not ask about it as much as they probably should. It is not going to warrant a syndrome, but that doesn't mean there isn't serious fallout from lack of sleep pretty quickly, both physiologically and psychologically. Moods head south and a brain that works quickly and efficiently becomes slow and muddled. It is a little inside joke in my family when I go to teach my

Sleep Deprivation

neuropsychology class about the brain without a workable one myself.

I have learned how to nurse myself through the particularly rough patches when it is worse than normal, or when I am not doing well emotionally (and usually the two go together). I have learned how to breathe and pray my way back to health, and to cancel the occasional class if I have to. I have rearranged my life and spend a good deal of my days recovering from my nights. I have made it as survivable as possible, and for the most part I am amazed at the resiliency of the human body.

But I blame this aspect of the disease for draining me of what used to be a brighter, more energetic personality with an easy sense of humor. And I blame the lack of sleep for holding me in its vice grip day after day, threatening to tip the scales of my own health if I don't honor it and work my entire life around it.

Maybe you have to find your own way, but my advice is to start compensating now. There is a cumulative effect of this disease and if I could do it over I would have incorporated restorative counterbalance to it earlier. You will probably have to change a great deal of your life to do so. Take up a practice that honors psychic balance and self-care—yoga, meditation, tai chi, or another martial art. Quit trying to do everything perfectly. Honor the sleep gods who are trying to keep you well. Let them have their way and don't fight them as long as I did. You're not going to win.

Impermanence

I started yoga in a pretty bad place. We were several years in and I was wearing down from the daily care. Psychologically, I was entering a phase where I could no longer deny facing his future directly like I could when it was newer and he was younger.

Sleep Deprivation

Rob and I were in individual survival mode and had lost our sense of solidarity that had gotten us through the first couple of years. The problem with having a child who needs extra or specific care of any kind is that you and your partner, if you are lucky enough to have one, become each other's relief. If one is exhausted or craves a few days off, the extra falls to the other. In order to relax and lighten up, your partner must become more stressed. You are never well-rested at the same time. You do not feel fun and light at the same time, together. Interactions become more like nursing reports than intimacy: "Ty was 340 about a half hour ago, bolused 3.2 units for it. What did he have for dinner? A little pasta so he might go high, but he's been running low on me at night. Pretty active today." Am I turning you on?

The fatigue had taken up residence in my body and manifested itself as pain, in my neck mostly. A lot of it stemmed from pushing myself ahead, thinking I could still exercise in the way I used to on the amount of sleep I was getting. I could still

The Superman Years

do everything I used to (I told myself), as if life hadn't changed completely and the same things would still work.

Actually, there was not much I could still do that I used to. The running I had consistently done since high school, which energized me physically and calmed me psychologically, now felt depleting and injurious, like it was harming my lower back and pulling on my neck in an uncomfortable way. This added depletion to depletion.

I knew I was producing some constant stress hormones, cortisol being chief among them (which ironically places one at risk for diabetes). I thought I might get sick myself if I found no way to replenish, and then what? Rattling around in my psyche at night was the thought, *if I go down, it leaves it all to Rob, by himself.* It's not a one-man job, although I know people do it alone. I don't know how, but they do. For me, it's all I can do to hang on with all the advantages I have: my own health, a partner, a fully involved partner, relative intelligence to figure

96

out the doses and other complexities of the care, and health insurance. I know people do it without help, but for our family, if one of us goes down, we leave the other with too much.

My own mental health was fluctuating with his blood sugar and believe me, it was a lot of getting "thrown around" psychologically. When I actually got myself down on a mat versus just reading about the philosophy of yoga, it was because I couldn't deal with the daily emotional thrashing. To make it long-term, I knew I needed to become more steadfast here and not be psychologically affected by every number on the screen ten times a day, up and down.

So I entered the practice in earnest. I needed this to "work." I worried though, that I would never again be as fit as I was "pre-diabetes," and that it would be a slow physical decline from there.

Initially I approached yoga like I had every other physical pursuit—push hard and force it to happen. I would just kind of put myself in the position of the pose, not really feeling the movement toward the pose or when my muscles were straining. I took classes with dancers, and even contortionists, and these were the models I used to emulate. Humility soon followed this ridiculous effort.

It took me a long time to even get close to the breathing of yoga. I had always held my breath through exertion before — here, you breathed. And if you couldn't, you backed off on the effort. This was a radical approach. I felt like I was gasping for air when I tried to breathe deep, like there was no way there would be enough, but I kept practicing and eventually I was able to breathe more deeply and easily. That's when I started to notice a change.

Now more attuned to the sensations in my body, instead of just plowing through the routine, I could more easily ascertain its needs. I could decide when it was most nurturing to hold back, and when it would be energizing to step it up. Some days—many days—lying flat on my back with my palms up in a receptive gesture is the most strengthening thing I can do for myself. It took me a long time to understand that though. The end result of slowing down is that paradoxically I've enjoyed the greatest physical strength of my life, perhaps because there is muscle restoration and surrender balanced with the exertion in yoga, which taught me something about how to deal with the caregiving required of diabetes.

And even though almost everyone has seen me cry (because I do it so easily now), I am actually much stronger emotionally than before diabetes because now I know how everything changes. Any difficult struggle is transient and will pass. Practicing yoga helped me enliven and lift the tissues and breathe vibrant air back into tight places that hadn't seen any air for awhile. Once re-exposed to oxygen, sheets of heat rippled down my shoulder blades and the pain greatly diminished. It allowed the fear, worry, and concern to move through me versus stagnate in my cells. I credit yoga for keeping me well.

The Superman Years

Mind states and outlooks don't stay the same from one minute to the next—not exactly the same anyway. Even a suicidal person who sees no other option can have a radical change of heart in the space of a beat.

There is an amazing story in a suicide documentary I show my students, *The Bridge*, told by a college student who is one of the rare survivors of a jump off the Golden Gate Bridge. The second his hands left the rails, he saw everything clearly and truthfully and wanted desperately to live. The problem was he was in the midst of a four second head-first free fall when he made this decision. He said he was *directed* how to turn and twist his position in the air so that when he broke the water at 120 mph, he did so with his boots first and landed as if sitting in a chair, thereby saving his life, but still managing to shatter his lower lumbar into splinters that tore into several organs.

He surfaced only to feel what he thought was a shark bumping about his feet and legs. He later learned it was a seal, keeping him afloat above the surface until he was rescued. This young man, Kevin, is a powerful mental health advocate now, letting people know suicide is never the right option.

Everything is just a moment. If I'm completely in my anxiety, lost and unable to find my way out of it, I know it will be different, even in five minutes. If I'm so tired I can't see straight, I will get some sleep at some point and everything will become more clear and less ominous. It will not be my permanent state.

Even Ty's blood sugar crises pass with amazing suddenness. We can be fretting and contemplating taking him to the hospital during a bout with the stomach flu, riding that cusp, and then the insulin takes, his blood sugar drops, he resurrects and is fine again just as if his life didn't hang in the balance an hour ago. Impermanence.

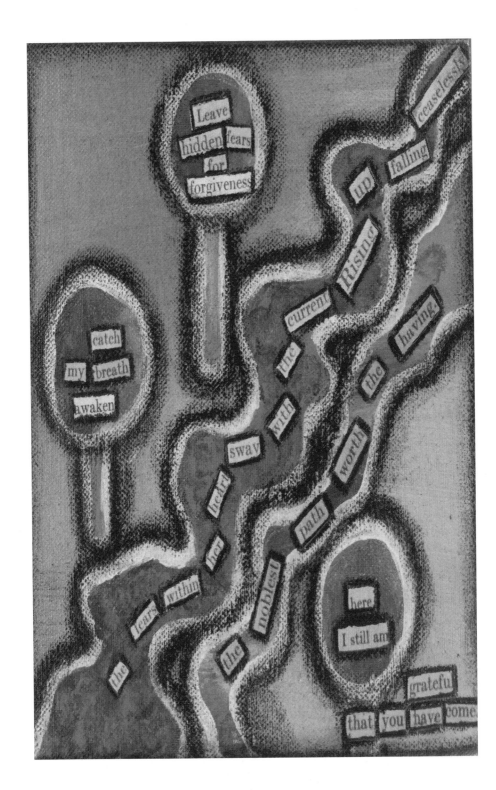

Chapter 5

Imagination

When the soul wishes to experience something she throws an image of the experience out before her and enters into her own image.

~ medieval mystic Meister Eckhart

The more mystical traditions in psychology talk about the realm of the imagination. Not imagination as in fantasy (something you're making up), more like dreaming while awake, except you don't command the storyline any more than you do in your night dreams. Instead, the images arise naturally in the psyche and reveal themselves to you.

The imagination has a rich history as part of visionary experiences in many ancient religious/spiritual traditions. It is thought of as an intermediate realm of images, dreams, impressions, and sensations which allows a line of communication with a deeper aspect of ourselves that is less available through the noise of our day-to-day activities. Think of it as a liminal place between two worlds—two aspects of ourselves. I'll describe it as the place that science cannot explain. It is a place of healing, and spontaneous remissions, and huge turnarounds the doctors were not expecting. They happen all the time. A place above the physical, containing knowledge beyond our five senses. My diagnosis dream probably came from this part of the psyche.

Images which appear in our mind and in our dreams are more powerful than most of us have been taught. They have a biological link to the physical reactions in the body, as they can invoke great emotion into it. We can all think of a dream that cranked out loads of adrenaline, or induced an orgasm, or left us emotionally hungover (good or bad), much of the next day.

Imagination

It's one of the reasons techniques such as guided imagery and creative visualization create change, especially visualizations involving biological and physical processes. Mentally practicing your tennis swing or sinking free throws markedly improves performance. The brain makes little distinction between imagining something and actually performing the action. I think visualizing might have been the reason Ty required so little insulin longer than his doctors expected.

Diabetes is considered an autoimmune disorder, meaning the immune system, for reasons not understood, destroys the insulin-producing cells in the pancreas. By the time symptoms arrive — the thirst and urination, weight loss and lethargy — sugar has built up in the blood stream because it can't get into the cells (where it is needed for sustenance), without the insulin to unlock them. By diagnosis, depending on the case, usually only about a quarter of functioning insulin-producing cells remain.

But what a difference that one quarter makes. It's so much harder to regulate blood sugar when it is gone. Researchers are working on finding ways to increase the lifespan of whatever functioning insulin-producing cells a person has left, and what wouldn't we all give for that? Who knows what we could stave off if we could prolong that little bit of natural functioning. In Ty's early years, we had no clinical choice but to let whatever insulin production just go away and die. That was hard to take.

Without a medical intervention, we decided to try something a little unconventional. At the time, Ty had an admiration and natural inclination toward all things militia. Where he got it I don't know, but the boy would fight anything with a gun, so that was the imagery we used. I suggested that at night when he's relaxed, laying in bed, that he imagine himself leading an army of healthy insulin-producing cells to fight off the damaging cells. I coached him through the first couple of nights, then left him on his own.

Imagination

Long after I had forgotten about the exercise, Ty's doc told me at a routine appointment that Ty continued to amaze the staff with his low dose of insulin relative to years out of diagnosis, indicating he was still producing some of his own. On the way home I asked Ty if he was still imagining the visualization. He told me he pictured it many nights.

I cannot prove empirically that the imagery is the reason Ty maintained cell functioning unusually long, but I would suggest it is certainly worth a harmless try. Use any imagery which speaks to your child. If you have a delicate, pink and purple princess, don't brandish her imagination with an AK 47. You might suggest she simply surround her healthy cells with a brilliant, impenetrable shield (in the color of her choice — purple? pink?). Better yet, let your child decide the appropriate image, perhaps an image she has been dreaming about. It's a simple technique with no ill side effects or invasive procedures.

Imaginary Scenarios

Fear automatically causes one type of picture to form in your mind, faith another. By virtue of learning how to handle the potential emergencies of this disease, you have to imagine scary scenes. In order to know how to deal with a bad low, for example, you have to picture yourself bringing your child out of it. When you learn about the possible complications over time, your mind, at some point, has to go down that path. It really can't be avoided.

I have spent a large portion of the last twelve years in the emotion of worry and fear. And knowing what I know about the power of images, I then meta-worried that the pictures in my head might bend or warp something in such a way that I may inadvertently be steering the future right into the scenario I feared.

Imagination

Simply becoming more conscious of the rampant thoughts in my brain helped me with this. Oftentimes, running on the autopilot of fear, we are unaware of what's playing through our minds. A high reading on the meter can play out as a lost toe by the time you jump in the shower. So first, we have to become aware that fear is ruling the psyche. This requires getting quiet on a regular basis. See what's there, playing out unconsciously in your head. What road is it going down? This creates some space in your mind and gives you more choice about how involved you want to be with the storyline, how true it is, and how much you want to be emotionally affected by it.

Then come back to what's true now — simply a high reading on the meter. He is OK now. You gave the insulin for the high. Recheck in an hour and a half and hope it is down — if not, give more. What else can you do? It's useless to jump ahead. It will not be the truth. This will create a much different effect on your body and mind than the false scenarios automatically generated by fear.

The Superman Years

Now I'm not telling you that if you are fearful you will cause bad things to happen, or that you shouldn't be scared, or that you're wrong to be scared—not at all. The emotion of fear is as natural as the earth and sky. I'm not of the mindset that with a little positive thinking all will be well and we'll all be rich. I'm still really scared a lot of the time and let's be real, we have a lot of things to be scared about.

alarm ever on

I
will never be
at ease or fearless

But I have confidence
from the long battle.
I will keep my son alive

gather your strength
draw your power

march forth and triumph

and how her fear at last was softened by sweet experience.

Chapter 6

Seizure

I feared it—feared it like no other. Other scary realities could be put off for awhile, but this you had to know how to deal with from Day One. If blood sugar goes too low too fast, or if it stays low too long, the person may become pale or glassy-eyed. He or she may act either unusually silly (punch drunk), or angry and agitated. They may sweat profusely, shake, or slump to the ground unresponsive. If the brain continues to be deprived of sugar for say, maybe another ten minutes, a person may seize or go unconscious; all thanks to the medicine which saves them.

I heard about it way too soon and way before I was ready to face it. A mother I met at the doctor's office the day of Ty's diagnosis called me to see how I was doing. The diagnosis was still new (just a few months in). We must have gotten on the scary topic of low blood sugar and in the course of the conversation she told me her daughter had had several seizures and that they were very hard to watch. I was not ready to hear it. "Nope," I said curtly to myself. "No, no, no, no, no," I mouthed as I shook my head and looked out the window. This will not happen. I will not let it. Even so, I practiced and practiced in my mind what to do in case of a bad low. I would guide juice down his throat if he could swallow, but if his throat was constricted by contractions, I would draw up the glucagon shot and stick it deep in his thigh. I would do it if I had to.

Glucagon is a concentrated sugar shot that comes in a bright red emergency kit with a needle about triple the thickness and length of his daily insulin syringes—long enough to reach the muscle—and a vial of sugary powder. It is a two-step process where you gently swirl the powder with liquid for twenty seconds to mix it, then draw the solution into the syringe. I wondered, should I ever have to use it, how would I ever be able to manage shaking hands through these steps as calmly and quickly as possible while my toddler convulsed upstairs, knowing I had to punch this large needle deep into his thigh? Would I remember how to do it? Would I be able to do it? I really hoped I would never have to do it.

Most severe lows happen at night, so I slept always just under the surface, almost as if I were not sleeping at all, as part of my consciousness was always on alert for it, like radar. And then one night I heard it. I sat upright in bed to a sound never present in my house before—a high pitched, rhythmic crying. I knew instantly it was happening and leapt into his room without thought. What I saw made me wince with sadness. Ty was shaking under the "S" emblem on the chest of his pajamas, and crying, except when the contractions squeezed his throat quiet. He appeared wide-eyed and scared. I forced myself to put my immediate reaction aside.

I remembered what my friend, Craig, had told me once about his own seizures and altered states. He told me Ty would likely not remember much about them. He would not be as traumatized as he appeared. The adrenaline that's released to exert sugar from the liver and muscle causes the dilated-eye, frightened look. The crying would just be a physiological reaction. He won't actually be sad, or scared, and he will not be in pain. Once his blood sugar hits eighty-four or so, he'll be fine. He might have a headache.

All these thoughts in the single stride across his room to his bedside where I scooped him up and told him, "It's OK baby, you're OK. We're going to get you some juice." I went into some sort of auto pilot I didn't know I had.

I fled with him down the stairs to the kitchen. We didn't keep juice in his room in those days, which seems funny to me now. I held him on the counter with one arm while finagling the straw wrapper with the other. I glanced at the clock on the microwave as I did so, making a mental note that I would call 911 if he didn't begin to come to in five minutes. First I'd try the juice.

Seizure

I managed to slowly work a box into him by carefully squirting it in small amounts down his throat between contractions. It is not medically advised to introduce anything into the mouth during a seizure, but it is the choice I made in the moment.

It worked. Within five minutes, the contractions softened and the time between them became discernibly lengthened. The crying stopped and only silent, regular shudders remained.

"He's coming out of it," I told Rob. My husband had heard noise and figured out what was happening. I didn't know what he was doing but I was aware of his presence moving quickly around me in the kitchen.

I scooted Ty to the edge of the counter against me, wrapped my arms full on around him and opened the palms of my hands wide and flat against his back. I wanted as much full-body contact as possible, so when he came back to normal awareness he would not be scared. After a few more minutes, Ty at last took a long, relaxed breath in. With the out breath, a final shiver rippled down the length of his back under the skin of my hands and out of his body at the base of his spine.

The sadness I had suppressed from earlier returned right then. Tears sprung to my eyes as we rested there, heads on each other's shoulders. I took a look at his face. He looked a little worn out and still glassy-eyed. "How you doing, kiddo?" I asked him. He just sighed and nodded his head. I hugged him again and said, "Let's go upstairs, huh?"

It was 4:30 am. I looked around the kitchen and then at Rob before turning off the light. From the looks of things, my guess is that what Rob was doing was opening and closing each and every cupboard and drawer looking for sugar in with the pots and the pans and the forks where we keep it. It looked like a giant wind had blown through.

"I get to sleep in your bed?" Ty asked, pleasantly surprised when we tossed him on our bed. He hopped across it, crawled under the covers with a smile on his face, and promptly fell back asleep like nothing had happened. Rob and I lied there, however, staring straight up at the ceiling like deer in headlights. I pulled the covers back. "Coffee?" I asked. Rob nodded.

***

I'd like to tell you that was it, our singular incident, but there have been others with varying degrees of consciousness altering. One time he had a freakishly low low at school. I spoke to him on the phone—clearly it was a close one. He was belligerent. The blood sugar was altering him and it unnerved me and brought me to my next fear—Ty going down at school in front of his friends. It has not happened though.

Another time we caught him at a dangerously low number on the meter (34), before he showed any symptoms. We plied him with juice, sat on either side of him on the couch and waited. He lost his vision and a single convulsion shuddered through him before the juice kicked.

A couple of times he hallucinated. He was old enough now that when he was able to talk and think coherently, I asked what he remembered of the experience. He said the closet doors spun all around each other and raced around the room in circles. He was most upset about the changing proportion of the juice box I kept shoving toward his face. It looked giant and scary and he was clearly still mad at me for it. "Don't ever do that again, Mom," he told me. I chuckled and told him I could not guarantee that.

I never have had to use the glucagon in twelve years. It still sits on a cool, dark shelf in our armoire, but I've been lax about keeping it fresh and unexpired. It's been ages since I've mentally practiced running through the steps of using it. Since I haven't needed it in all this time, I sit in false comfort that I never will. This is irrational, however, as I know the possibility exists at all times. It could just as easily be tonight as years down the road.

It's not like we'll ever be out of the woods, anytime.

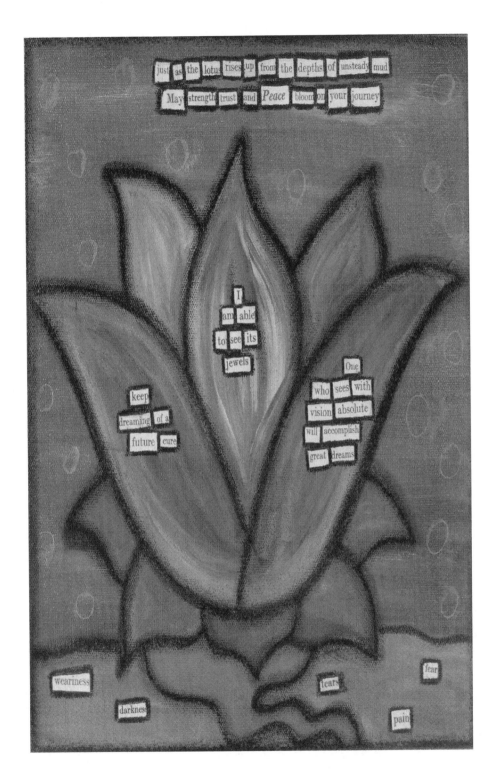

Chapter 7

Vision

Keep on dreaming, it's never too late

Keep on dreaming, cause that's what it take

~Ziggy Marley

Before and After

I sometimes wonder how my life would have gone without it. What kind of person I would be and what I would be doing. What would my marriage be like if diabetes hadn't come into our lives?

I can tell you, I'm glad for it. In those respects, I'm glad for it. Don't get me wrong, I'd give anything for Ty not to have it, but in many ways these have been the best years of my life. I know I wouldn't be writing this book. I probably would not teach on the topics I do, teach in the way I do, or emphasize the things I do.

As for my marriage? Hard to say what would have become of us and what kind of people we would have turned into without the help the disease gave to take us where we both wanted. I can tell you it took a wholehearted willingness on both our parts to let the pre-diabetes "us" go completely. Why we made it and so many don't I cannot even say—by some grace.

Jalyn, the quiet, sensitive one I felt so sorry for, now drives and dislikes me often. Ty got a lot of attention over the years for his diabetes and got asked a lot of questions, which he seemed to relish. This seemed to suit Jalyn just fine. She seemed content to stay in the background, happy not to have it. She shows Ty no sympathies but treats him like the little brother he is—as it should be.

Vision

Ty is nearly fifteen now. You would never know he has a life-threatening disease by looking at him. You can't tell from the outside the daunting daily reality that keeps him afloat. He appears healthy and whole, and physically fit, thankfully. He is his father's son in that he is maniacally active. You'd never guess and I am glad. The only downside being that it tends to lead to false assumptions from the general population that his diabetes is not serious.

His room is no longer red and blue of course. The walls have been replaced with equally obnoxious green and gold (an ode to the Green Bay Packers), thanks to no small indoctrination effort on the part of my husband. The kid was born and raised in Colorado but taught to shun the Denver Broncos at an early age. He wore Packer stuff amid the sea of Broncos jerseys in all his classrooms. He lived the glorious Favre years and watched a winning playoff game at Lambeau field in a snowstorm, all the while cheering and having the best time. So Superman has been incognito for many years, but I resisted painting over those bright red and blue walls. I knew it meant the end of an era—superpowers going undercover.

Ty remembers little of the bad lows from his early childhood, and the teenager in him only half-believes what I say could happen if he doesn't check his blood sugar regularly. We have entered a phase where he has to find his own edges, his own truths. His diabetes is not mine.

As such he will take it over—all of it. It breaks my heart to think of what will become his in the next few years as he transitions through high school to college and life on his own. One day this fatigue and exhaustion may be his to bear, factors which will only intensify rapidly fluctuating blood sugar.

I hope we are able to give it to him in a way which promotes lifelong balance, not punishing rigidity, and that we have prepared him for the long term. Recently, after catching him at a random and dangerous low number in the middle of the night, I said to him apologetically the next morning, "You know Ty, when you're on your own . . . you're going to have to check. I don't think you're going to be able to make it through the nights without checking." He said sincerely, "I know Mom," as if he had given it some previous thought. I was sorry for him, picturing him in a college dorm room, trying to take care of himself in that context. My hope is that the Superman qualities are merely under the surface and can be called upon when needed, when the day to day is overwhelming, or when there is a crisis in the dead of night.

Facing Future

I caught my friend Michael J. Fox unexpectedly on CNN recently, just as I sat folding the laundry one day while struggling with my stance on hope. I hadn't seen him in awhile and I was glad to. He was right there with Christopher Reeve, speaking for me, when he didn't have to be. Although it must have taken a Herculean effort to appear, he didn't let a few full-body dyskinesias keep him from speaking on the impact of medical research on his life, twenty-plus years into his progressive illness. Throughout the interview he never failed to affirm his belief and focus on a cure for Parkinson's disease. If Michael holds steadfast and does not waver as he lives the life, who am I to?

I try to hold steadfast to a dream I had not long after Ty's diagnosis, where I took him to the clinic, as I did in his diagnosis dream. This time, though, they injected healthy cells into his side through a long syringe as he sat there watching and smiling. He hopped off the table and that was it. The healthy cells took over and he forever after produced his own insulin again. I felt it, that elation, as if it were true.

I hope this dream to come true. If I had my way, the cure would be here and this book would be reflecting on his years with diabetes. I know we, or a future generation of parents, are going to look back on this one day and say to each other, "Can you believe the things we used to have to do? How ridiculous and archaic our daily routine was?" I wish that day were now.

I beg to be relieved by the cure. But if that is not yet to be, I ask for strength for our families to withstand the burden despite the rigorous daily care, the chronic sleep deprivation, and the deep emotions of grief, through learning to live without control, without absolutes, without answers, or a timeline on a cure. Despite no relief, no assurance, no comfort, I ask that we remain strong and uplifted in our belief.

And there among the fearful images you might hold about the future, I ask you to imagine it differently. Dream your own version of my dream. Picture your child being cured by any means you believe possible. Plan your happy celebration where you burn your supplies. I can be a pretty foolish idealist, but really, can you feel this?

Hold that image among the rest at all times and allow the feeling it engenders. Remember it often at your most despairing moments.

Go ahead and send them to me, your imaginings, and I will show you the collective force in them—the hopes of parents with kids who suffer. And I trust that something about our common envisioning will change things, move things forward in the way we have imagined, wished fervently for, dreamed of- toward healing you and your child whether or not there is insulin-dependence.

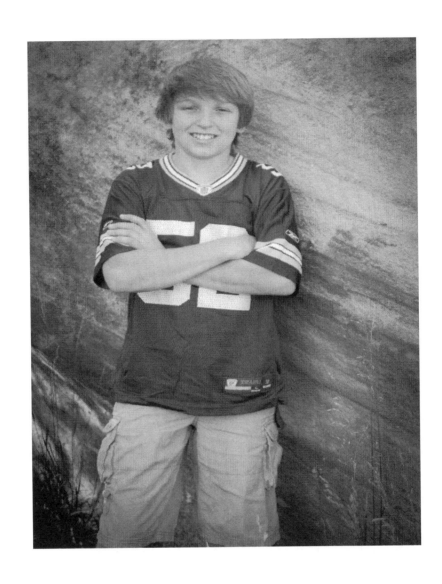

Older Superman

Acknowledgements:

Rob, Jalyn, and Ty, you are everything to me. I'm so grateful we are in this together. Thank you for putting up with an unstable mood, abnormal isolation, and a preoccupied mind during the long months of writing. To my first and last reader, Rob, whose feedback was invaluable on so many levels, thank you, and I love you. Jalyn and Ty, thanks for bringing me out of my intensity by needing mundane things and demanding to still be fed.

All these years we have been sustained by a grace called family and dear friends who showed us compassion, grieved with us, celebrated with us, and helped us with the care. We were never alone. You mean the world to us. Much gratitude to our parents, Don and Jeanette Rupnow, and Phyllis and William Buzogany. I'm sure it has been no emotional picnic worrying about Rob and I in the same way we worry about Ty.

Susan Upson and Ann Stark, how would I ever have made it without you? Thank you for your never-ending care of Ty through the Superman/Packer years at school. I never would have been able to write without the peace of mind you provided.

Thank you to Bob Weisenberg, Associate Publisher at Elephant Journal and my dear friend, for the confidence, encouragement, and praise of my writing, and for being the one to bring it into the public realm for actual people to read. Jeff Raff, thank you for your kind words in the foreword of this book, but more so, for all I have learned from you about dreams and the inner life, and for all the immeasurable ways you have helped me. To my brother, Larry Rupnow, thank you for making me climb a mountain I wasn't sure I could climb, literally and figuratively, and for taking a huge load off by allowing me to dump, I mean, by "offering" to take on the more detailed work of this project I just couldn't face. Kathryn Adler-Kath, thank you for providing the amazing artwork in these pages I know was born out of your own pain, and for being my creative touchstone and true friend for the past twenty-five or so years. Each of you made my writing better in a different way.

Gregg Mangan! Thank you for agreeing to join the ride and guide a first-time author through the editing process. I loved the way you took the reins just when I needed someone who knew what they were doing. It has been an adventure I treasure, and I will not hesitate to seek out your professionalism in the future. Di, my sister, thanks for the creativity and logistics you endured in creating the cover art as only you could do. Dr. Peggy Norwood, Terri Lukavitch, and Lara Wells, you supported, encouraged, and cheerleaded when it was just an idea. Thank you.

To James Altucher, my writing buddy at Elephant Journal, I'm indebted. No James, no book. Simple as that.

Gratitude to Barb, Terri, and Jacqueline Bendrick who allowed their difficult story to be told here. And to the Creases, for being such great friends to us all the way along this difficult, joyous road.

About The Author:

Linda Buzogany is a professor of psychology and a licensed professional counselor. She currently teaches classes on neuropsychology, dreams and consciousness, and abnormal psychology. Prior to teaching, Linda worked as a therapist in inpatient psychiatric hospitals. Contact: buzco@aol.com.

Made in the USA
Middletown, DE
23 November 2015